Table of Contents

CW00516122

DASH DIET COOKBOOK

2021

HEALTHY RECIPES TO LOWER BLOOD PRESSURE

SARAH JOHNSON

Chicken and Lentils Mix

Preparation time: 10 minutes
Cooking time: 25 minutes
Servings: 4

Ingredients:
- 1 cup canned tomatoes, no-salt-added, chopped
- Black pepper to the taste
- 1 tablespoon chipotle paste
- 1 pound chicken breast, skinless, boneless and cubed
- 2 cups canned lentils, no-salt-added, drained and rinsed
- ½ tablespoon olive oil
- 1 yellow onion, chopped
- 2 tablespoons cilantro, chopped

Directions:
1. Heat up a pan with the oil over medium heat, add the onion and chipotle paste, stir and sauté for 5 minutes.
2. Add the chicken, toss and brown for 5 minutes.
3. Add the rest of the ingredients, toss, cook everything for 15 minutes, divide into bowls and serve.

Nutrition: calories 369, fat 17.6, fiber 9, carbs 44.8, protein 23.5

Chicken and Cauliflower

Preparation time: 5 minutes
Cooking time: 25 minutes
Servings: 4

Ingredients:
- 1 pound chicken breast, skinless, boneless and cubed
- 2 cups cauliflower florets
- 1 tablespoon olive oil
- 1 red onion, chopped
- 1 tablespoon balsamic vinegar
- ½ cup red bell pepper, chopped
- A pinch of black pepper
- 2 garlic cloves, minced
- ½ cup low-sodium chicken stock
- 1 cup canned tomatoes, no-salt-added, chopped

Directions:
1. Heat up a pan with the oil over medium-high heat, add the onion, garlic and the meat and brown for 5 minutes.
2. Add the rest of the ingredients, toss and cook over medium heat for 20 minutes.
3. Divide everything into bowls and serve for lunch.

Nutrition: calories 366, fat 12, fiber 5.6, carbs 44.3, protein 23.7

Basil Tomato and Carrots Soup

Preparation time: 10 minutes
Cooking time: 20 minutes
Servings: 4

Ingredients:
- 3 garlic cloves, minced
- 1 yellow onion, chopped
- 3 carrots, chopped
- 1 tablespoon olive oil
- 20 ounces roasted tomatoes, no-salt-added
- 2 cup low-sodium veggie stock
- 1 tablespoon basil, dried
- 1 cup coconut cream
- A pinch of black pepper

Directions:
1. Heat up a pot with the oil over medium heat, add the onion and the garlic and sauté for 5 minutes.
2. Add the rest of the ingredients, stir, bring to a simmer, cook for 15 minutes, blend the soup using an immersion blender, divide into bowls and serve for lunch.

Nutrition: calories 244, fat 17.8, fiber 4.7, carbs 18.6, protein 3.8

Pork with Sweet Potatoes

Preparation time: 10 minutes
Cooking time: 30 minutes
Servings: 4

Ingredients:
- 4 pork chops, boneless
- 1 pound sweet potatoes, peeled and cut into wedges
- 1 tablespoon olive oil
- 1 cup vegetable stock, low-sodium
- A pinch of black pepper
- 1 teaspoon oregano, dried
- 1 teaspoon rosemary, dried
- 1 teaspoon basil, dried

Directions:
1. Heat up a pan with the oil over medium-high heat, add the pork chops and cook them for 4 minutes on each side.
2. Add the sweet potatoes and the rest of the ingredients, put the lid on and cook over medium heat for 20 minutes more stirring from time to time.
3. Divide everything between plates and serve.

Nutrition: calories 424, fat 23.7, fiber 5.1, carbs 32.3, protein 19.9

Trout and Carrots Soup

Preparation time: 10 minutes
Cooking time: 25 minutes
Servings: 4

Ingredients:

- 1 yellow onion, chopped
- 12 cups low-sodium fish stock
- 1 pound carrots, sliced
- 1 pound trout fillets, boneless, skinless and cubed
- 1 tablespoon sweet paprika
- 1 cup tomatoes, cubed
- 1 tablespoon olive oil
- Black pepper to the taste

Directions:

1. Heat up a pot with the oil over medium-high heat, add the onion, stir and sauté for 5 minutes.
2. Add the fish, carrots and the rest of the ingredients, bring to a simmer and cook over medium heat for 20 minutes.
3. Ladle the soup into bowls and serve.

Nutrition: calories 361, fat 13.4, fiber 4.6, carbs 164, protein 44.1

Turkey and Fennel Stew

Preparation time: 10 minutes
Cooking time: 45 minutes
Servings: 4

Ingredients:
- 1 turkey breast, skinless, boneless and cubed
- 2 fennel bulbs, sliced
- 1 tablespoon olive oil
- 2 bay leaves
- 1 yellow onion, chopped
- 1 cup canned tomatoes, no-salt-added
- 2 low-sodium beef stock
- 3 garlic cloves, chopped
- Black pepper to the taste

Directions:
1. Heat up a pan with the oil over medium heat, add the onion and the meat and brown for 5 minutes.
2. Add the fennel and the rest of the ingredients, bring to a simmer and cook over medium heat for 40 minutes, stirring from time to time.
3. Divide the stew into bowls and serve.

Nutrition: calories 371, fat 12.8, fiber 5.3, carbs 16.7, protein 11.9

Eggplant Soup

Preparation time: 10 minutes
Cooking time: 30 minutes
Servings: 4

Ingredients:
- 2 big eggplants, roughly cubed
- 1 quart low-sodium veggie stock
- 2 tablespoons no-salt-added tomato paste
- 1 red onion, chopped
- 1 tablespoon olive oil
- 1 tablespoon cilantro, chopped
- A pinch of black pepper

Directions:
1. Heat up a pot with the oil over medium heat, add the onion, stir and sauté for 5 minutes.
2. Add the eggplants and the other ingredients, bring to a simmer over medium heat, cook for 25 minutes, divide into bowls and serve.

Nutrition: calories 335, fat 14.4, fiber 5, carbs 16.1, protein 8.4

Sweet Potatoes Cream

Preparation time: 10 minutes
Cooking time: 25 minutes
Servings: 4

Ingredients:

- 4 cups veggie stock
- 2 tablespoons avocado oil
- 2 sweet potatoes, peeled and cubed
- 2 yellow onions, chopped
- 2 garlic cloves, minced
- 1 cup coconut milk
- A pinch of black pepper
- ½ teaspoon basil, chopped

Directions:

1. Heat up a pot with the oil over medium heat, add the onion and the garlic, stir and sauté for 5 minutes.
2. Add the sweet potatoes and the rest of the ingredients, bring to a simmer and cook over medium heat for 20 minutes.
3. Blend the soup using an immersion blender, ladle into bowls and serve for lunch.

Nutrition: calories 303, fat 14.4, fiber 4, carbs 9.8, protein 4.5

Chicken and Mushrooms Soup

Preparation time: 10 minutes
Cooking time: 30 minutes
Servings: 4

Ingredients:

- 1 quart veggie stock, low-sodium
- 1 tablespoon ginger, grated
- 1 yellow onion, chopped
- 1 tablespoon olive oil
- 1 pound chicken breast, skinless, boneless and cubed
- ½ pound white mushrooms, sliced
- 4 Thai chilies, chopped
- ¼ cup lime juice
- ¼ cup cilantro, chopped
- A pinch of black pepper

Directions:

1. Heat up a pot with the oil over medium heat, add the onion, ginger, chilies and the meat, stir and brown for 5 minutes.
2. Add the mushrooms, stir and cook for 5 minutes more.
3. Add the rest of the ingredients, bring to a simmer and cook over medium heat for 20 minutes more.
4. Ladle the soup into bowls and serve right away.

Nutrition: calories 226, fat 8.4, fiber 3.3, carbs 13.6, protein 28.2

Lime Salmon Pan

Preparation time: 10 minutes
Cooking time: 20 minutes
Servings: 4

Ingredients:
- 4 salmon fillet, boneless
- 3 garlic cloves, minced
- 1 yellow onion, chopped
- Black pepper to the taste
- 2 tablespoons olive oil
- Juice of 1 lime
- 1 tablespoon lime zest, grated
- 1 tablespoon thyme, chopped

Directions:
1. Heat up a pan with the oil over medium-high heat, add the onion and garlic, stir and sauté for 5 minutes.
2. Add the fish and cook it for 3 minutes on each side.
3. Add the rest of the ingredients, cook everything for 10 minutes more, divide between plates and serve for lunch.

Nutrition: calories 315, fat 18.1, fiber 1.1, carbs 4.9, protein 35.1

Potato Salad

Preparation time: 10 minutes
Cooking time: 20 minutes
Servings: 4

Ingredients:
- 2 tomatoes, chopped
- 2 avocados, pitted and chopped
- 2 cups baby spinach
- 2 scallions, chopped
- 1 pound gold potatoes, boiled, peeled and cut into wedges
- 1 tablespoon olive oil
- 1 tablespoon lemon juice
- 1 yellow onion, chopped
- 2 garlic cloves, minced
- Black pepper to the taste
- 1 bunch cilantro, chopped

Directions:
1. Heat up a pan with the oil over medium-high heat, add the onion, scallions and the garlic, stir and sauté for 5 minutes.
2. Add the potatoes, toss gently and cook for 5 minutes more.
3. Add the rest of the ingredients, toss, cook over medium heat for 10 minutes more, divide into bowls and serve for lunch.

Nutrition: calories 342, fat 23.4, fiber 11.7, carbs 33.5, protein 5

Ground Beef and Tomato Pan

Preparation time: 10 minutes
Cooking time: 20 minutes
Servings: 4

Ingredients:
- 1 pound beef, ground
- 1 red onion, chopped
- 1 tablespoon olive oil
- 1 cup cherry tomatoes, halved
- ½ red bell pepper, chopped
- Black pepper to the taste
- 1 tablespoon chives, chopped
- 1 tablespoon rosemary, chopped
- 3 tablespoons low-sodium beef stock

Directions:
1. Heat up a pan with the oil over medium heat, add the onion and the bell pepper, stir and sauté for 5 minutes.
2. Add the meat, stir and brown it for another 5 minutes.
3. Add the rest of the ingredients, toss, cook for 10 minutes, divide into bowls and serve for lunch.

Nutrition: calories 320, fat 11.3, fiber 4.4, carbs 18.4, protein 9

Shrimp and Avocado Salad

Preparation time: 5 minutes
Cooking time: 0 minutes
Servings: 4

Ingredients:
- 1 orange, peeled and cut into segments
- 1 pound shrimp, cooked, peeled and deveined
- 2 cups baby arugula
- 1 avocado, pitted, peeled and cubed
- 2 tablespoons olive oil
- 2 tablespoons balsamic vinegar
- Juice of ½ orange
- Salt and black pepper

Directions:
1. In a salad bowl, mix combine the shrimp with the oranges and the other ingredients, toss and serve for lunch.

Nutrition: calories 300, fat 5.2, fiber 2, carbs 11.4, protein 6.7

Broccoli Cream

Preparation time: 10 minutes
Cooking time: 40 minutes
Servings: 4

Ingredients:
- 2 pounds broccoli florets
- 1 yellow onion, chopped
- 1 tablespoon olive oil
- Black pepper to the taste
- 2 garlic cloves, minced
- 3 cups low-sodium beef stock
- 1 cup coconut milk
- 2 tablespoons cilantro, chopped

Directions:
1. Heat up a pot with the oil over medium heat, add the onion and the garlic, stir and sauté for 5 minutes.
2. Add the broccoli and the other ingredients except the coconut milk, bring to a simmer and cook over medium heat for 35 minutes more.
3. Blend the soup using an immersion blender, add the coconut milk, pulse again, divide into bowls and serve.

Nutrition: calories 330, fat 11.2, fiber 9.1, carbs 16.4, protein 9.7

Cabbage Soup

Preparation time: 10 minutes
Cooking time: 40 minutes
Servings: 4

Ingredients:
- 1 big green cabbage head, roughly shredded
- 1 yellow onion, chopped
- 1 tablespoon olive oil
- Black pepper to the taste
- 1 leek, chopped
- 2 cups canned tomatoes, low-sodium
- 4 cups chicken stock, low-sodium
- 1 tablespoon cilantro, chopped

Directions:
1. Heat up a pot with the oil over medium heat, add the onion and the leek, stir and cook for 5 minutes.
2. Add the cabbage and the rest of the ingredients except the cilantro, bring to a simmer and cook over medium heat for 35 minutes.
3. Ladle the soup into bowls, sprinkle the cilantro on top and serve.

Nutrition: calories 340, fat 11.7, fiber 6, carbs 25.8, protein 11.8

Celery and Cauliflower Soup

Preparation time: 10 minutes
Cooking time: 40 minutes
Servings: 4

Ingredients:

- 2 pounds cauliflower florets
- 1 red onion, chopped
- 1 tablespoon olive oil
- 1 cup tomato puree
- Black pepper to the taste
- 1 cup celery, chopped
- 6 cups low-sodium chicken stock
- 1 tablespoon dill, chopped

Directions:

4. Heat up a pot with the oil over medium-high heat, add the onion and the celery, stir and sauté for 5 minutes.
5. Add the cauliflower and the rest of the ingredients, bring to a simmer and cook over medium heat for 35 minutes more.
6. Divide the soup into bowls and serve.

Nutrition: calories 135, fat 4, fiber 8, carbs 21.4, protein 7.7

Pork and Leeks Soup

Preparation time: 10 minutes
Cooking time: 40 minutes
Servings: 4

Ingredients:

- 1 pound pork stew meat, cubed
- Black pepper to the taste
- 5 leeks, chopped
- 1 yellow onion, chopped
- 2 tablespoons olive oil
- 1 tablespoon parsley, chopped
- 6 cups low-sodium beef stock

Directions:

4. Heat up a pot with the oil over medium-high heat, add the onion and the leeks, stir and sauté for 5 minutes.
5. Add the meat, stir and brown for 5 minutes more.
6. Add the rest of the ingredients, bring to a simmer and cook over medium heat for 30 minutes.
7. Ladle the soup into bowls and serve.

Nutrition: calories 395, fat 18.3, fiber 2.6, carbs 18.4, protein 38.2

Minty Shrimp and Broccoli Salad

Preparation time: 5 minutes
Cooking time: 20 minutes
Servings: 4

Ingredients:

- 1/3 cup low-sodium veggie stock
- 2 tablespoons olive oil
- 2 cups broccoli florets
- 1 pound shrimp, peeled and deveined
- Black pepper to the taste
- 1 yellow onion, chopped
- 4 cherry tomatoes, halved
- 2 garlic cloves, minced
- Juice of ½ lemon
- ½ cup kalamata olives, pitted and cut into halves
- 1 tablespoon mint, chopped

Directions:

1. Heat up a pan with the oil over medium-high heat, add the onion and the garlic, stir and sauté for 3 minutes.
2. Add the shrimp, toss and cook for 2 minutes more.
3. Add the broccoli and the other ingredients, toss, cook everything for 10 minutes, divide into bowls and serve for lunch.

Nutrition: calories 270, fat 11.3, fiber 4.1, carbs 14.3, protein 28.9

Shrimp and Cod Soup

Preparation time: 10 minutes
Cooking time: 20 minutes
Servings: 4

Ingredients:

- 1 quart low-sodium chicken stock
- ½ pound shrimp, peeled and deveined
- ½ pound cod fillets, boneless, skinless and cubed
- 2 tablespoons olive oil
- 2 teaspoons chili powder
- 1 teaspoon sweet paprika
- 2 shallots, chopped
- A pinch of black pepper
- 1 tablespoon dill, chopped

Directions:

1. Heat up a pot with the oil over medium heat, add the shallots, stir and sauté for 5 minutes.
2. Add the shrimp and the cod, and cook for 5 minutes more.
3. Add the rest of the ingredients, bring to a simmer and cook over medium heat for 10 minutes.
4. Divide the soup into bowls and serve.

Nutrition: calories 189, fat 8.8, fiber 0.8, carbs 3.2, protein 24.6

Shrimp and Green Onions Mix

Preparation time: 10 minutes
Cooking time: 10 minutes
Servings: 4

Ingredients:
- 2 pounds shrimp, peeled and deveined
- 1 cup cherry tomatoes, halved
- 1 tablespoon olive oil
- 4 green onion, chopped
- 1 tablespoon balsamic vinegar
- 1 tablespoon chives, chopped

Directions:
1. Heat up a pan with the oil over medium heat, add the onion, and the cherry tomatoes, stir and sauté for 4 minutes.
2. Add the shrimp and the other ingredients, cook for 6 minutes more, divide between plates and serve.

Nutrition: calories 313, fat 7.5, fiber 1, carbs 6.4, protein 52.4

Spinach Stew

Preparation time: 10 minutes
Cooking time: 15 minutes
Servings: 4

Ingredients:
- 1 tablespoons olive oil
- 1 teaspoon ginger, grated
- 2 garlic cloves, minced
- 1 yellow onion, chopped
- 2 tomatoes, chopped
- 1 cup canned tomatoes, no-salt-added
- 1 teaspoon cumin, ground
- A pinch of black pepper
- 1 cup low-sodium veggie stock
- 2 pounds spinach leaves

Directions:
1. Heat up a pot with the oil over medium heat, add the ginger, garlic and the onion, stir and sauté for 5 minutes.
2. Add the tomatoes, canned tomatoes and the other ingredients, toss gently, bring to a simmer and cook for 10 minutes more.
3. Divide the stew into bowls and serve.

Nutrition: calories 123, fat 4.8, fiber 7.3, carbs 17, protein 8.2

Curry Cauliflower Mix

Preparation time: 10 minutes
Cooking time: 25 minutes
Servings: 4

Ingredients:
- 1 red onion, chopped
- 1 tablespoon olive oil
- 2 garlic cloves, minced
- 1 red bell pepper, chopped
- 1 green bell pepper, chopped
- 1 tablespoon lime juice
- 1 pound cauliflower florets
- 14 ounces canned tomatoes, chopped
- 2 teaspoons curry powder
- A pinch of black pepper
- 2 cups coconut cream
- 1 tablespoon cilantro, chopped

Directions:
1. Heat up a pot with the oil over medium heat, add the onion and the garlic, stir and cook for 5 minutes.
2. Add the bell peppers and the other ingredients, bring everything to a simmer and cook over medium heat for 20 minutes.
3. Divide everything into bowls and serve.

Nutrition: calories 270, fat 7.7, fiber 5.4, carbs 12.9, protein 7

Carrots and Zucchini Stew

Preparation time: 10 minutes
Cooking time: 30 minutes
Servings: 4

Ingredients:

- 1 yellow onion, chopped
- 2 tablespoons olive oil
- 2 garlic cloves, minced
- 4 zucchinis, sliced
- 2 carrots, sliced
- 1 teaspoon sweet paprika
- ¼ teaspoon chili powder
- A pinch of black pepper
- ½ cup tomatoes, chopped
- 2 cups low-sodium veggie stock
- 1 tablespoon chives, chopped
- 1 tablespoon rosemary, chopped

Directions:

1. Heat up a pot with the oil over medium heat, add the onion and the garlic, stir and sauté for 5 minutes.
2. Add the zucchinis, carrots and the other ingredients, bring to a simmer and cook for 25 minutes more.
3. Divide the stew in to bowls and serve right away for lunch.

Nutrition: calories 272, fat 4.6, fiber 4.7, carbs 14.9, protein 9

Cabbage and Green Beans Stew

Preparation time: 10 minutes
Cooking time: 25 minutes
Servings: 4

Ingredients:
- 2 tablespoons olive oil
- 1 red cabbage head, shredded
- 1 red onion, chopped
- 1 pound green beans, trimmed and halved
- 2 garlic cloves, minced
- 7 ounces canned tomatoes, no-salt-added chopped
- 2 cups low-sodium veggie stock
- A pinch of black pepper
- 1 tablespoon dill, chopped

Directions:
1. Heat up a pot with the oil, over medium heat, add the onion and the garlic, stir and sauté for 5 minutes.
2. Add the cabbage and the other ingredients, stir, cover and simmer over medium heat for 20 minutes.
3. Divide into bowls and serve for lunch.

Nutrition: calories 281, fat 8.5, fiber 7.1, carbs 14.9, protein 6.7

Chili Mushroom Soup

Preparation time: 5 minutes
Cooking time: 30 minutes
Servings: 4

Ingredients:

- 1 yellow onion, chopped
- 1 tablespoon olive oil
- 1 red chili pepper, chopped
- 1 teaspoon chili powder
- ½ teaspoon hot paprika
- 4 garlic cloves, minced
- 1 pound white mushrooms, sliced
- 6 cups low-sodium veggie stock
- 1 cup tomatoes, chopped
- ½ tablespoon parsley, chopped

Directions:

1. Heat up a pot with the oil, over medium heat, add the onion, chili pepper, hot paprika, chili powder and the garlic, stir and sauté for 5 minutes.
2. Add the mushrooms, stir and cook for 5 minutes more.
3. Add the rest of the ingredients, bring to a simmer and cook over medium heat for 20 minutes.
4. Divide the soup into bowls and serve.

Nutrition: calories 290, fat 6.6, fiber 4.6, carbs 16.9, protein 10

Chili Pork

Preparation time: 10 minutes
Cooking time: 30 minutes
Servings: 4

Ingredients:
- 2 pounds pork stew meat, cubed
- 2 tablespoons chili paste
- 1 yellow onion, chopped
- 2 garlic cloves, minced
- 1 tablespoon olive oil
- 2 cups low-sodium beef stock
- 1 tablespoon oregano, chopped

Directions:
1. Heat up a pot with the oil, over medium-high heat, add the onion and the garlic, stir and sauté for 5 minutes.
2. Add the meat and brown it for 5 minutes more.
3. Add the rest of the ingredients, bring to a simmer and cook over medium heat for 20 minutes more.
4. Divide the mix into bowls and serve.

Nutrition: calories 363, fat 8.6, fiber 7, carbs 17.3, protein 18.4

Paprika Mushroom and Salmon Salad

Preparation time: 10 minutes
Cooking time: 20 minutes
Servings: 4

Ingredients:
- 10 ounces smoked salmon, low-sodium, boneless, skinless and cubed
- 2 green onions, chopped
- 2 red chili peppers, chopped
- 1 tablespoon olive oil
- ½ teaspoon oregano, dried
- ½ teaspoon smoked paprika
- A pinch of black pepper
- 8 ounces white mushrooms, sliced
- 1 tablespoon lemon juice
- 1 cup black olives, pitted and halved
- 1 tablespoon parsley, chopped

Directions:
1. Heat up a pan with the oil over medium heat, add the onions and chili peppers, stir and cook for 4 minutes.
2. Add the mushrooms, stir and sauté them for 5 minutes.
3. Add the salmon and the other ingredients, toss, cook everything for 10 minutes more, divide into bowls and serve for lunch.

Nutrition: calories 321, fat 8.5, fiber 8, carbs 22.2, protein 13.5

Chickpeas and Potatoes Medley

Preparation time: 10 minutes
Cooking time: 30 minutes
Servings: 4

Ingredients:
- 2 tablespoons olive oil
- 1 cup canned chickpeas, no-salt-added, drained and rinsed
- 1 pound sweet potatoes, peeled and cut into wedges
- 4 garlic cloves, minced
- 2 shallots, chopped
- 1 cup canned tomatoes, no-salt-added and chopped
- 1 teaspoon coriander, ground
- 2 tomatoes, chopped
- 1 cup low-sodium veggie stock
- A pinch of black pepper
- 1 tablespoon lemon juice
- 1 tablespoon cilantro, chopped

Directions:
1. Heat up a pot with the oil over medium heat, add the shallots and the garlic, stir and sauté for 5 minutes.
2. Add the chickpeas, potatoes and the other ingredients, bring to a simmer and cook over medium heat for 25 minutes.
3. Divide everything into bowls and serve for lunch.

Nutrition: calories 341, fat 11.7, fiber 6, carbs 14.9, protein 18.7

Cardamom Chicken Mix

Preparation time: 10 minutes
Cooking time: 30 minutes
Servings: 4

Ingredients:

- 1 tablespoon olive oil
- 1 pound chicken breast, skinless, boneless and cubed
- 1 shallot, chopped
- 1 tablespoon ginger, grated
- 2 garlic cloves, minced
- 1 teaspoon cardamom, ground
- ½ teaspoon turmeric powder
- 1 teaspoon lime juice
- 1 cup low-sodium chicken stock
- 1 tablespoon cilantro, chopped

Directions:

1. Heat up a pot with the oil over medium-high heat, add the shallot, ginger, garlic, cardamom and the turmeric, stir and sauté for 5 minutes.
2. Add the meat and brown it for 5 minutes.
3. Add the rest of the ingredients, bring everything to a simmer and cook for 20 minutes.
4. Divide the mix into bowls and serve.

Nutrition: calories 175, fat 6.5, fiber 0.5, carbs 3.3, protein 24.7

Lentils Chili

Preparation time: 10 minutes
Cooking time: 35 minutes
Servings: 6

Ingredients:
- 1 green bell pepper, chopped
- 1 tablespoon olive oil
- 2 spring onions, chopped
- 2 garlic cloves, minced
- 24 ounces canned lentils, no-salt-added, drained and rinsed
- 2 cups veggie stock
- 2 tablespoons chili powder, mild
- ½ teaspoon chipotle powder
- 30 ounces canned tomatoes, no-salt-added, chopped
- A pinch of black pepper

Directions:
1. Heat up a pot with the oil over medium heat, add the onions and the garlic, stir and sauté for 5 minutes.
2. Add the bell pepper, lentils and the other ingredients, bring to a simmer and cook over medium heat for 30 minutes.
3. Divide the chili into bowls and serve for lunch.

Nutrition: calories 466, fat 5, fiber 37.6, carbs 77.9, protein 31.2

Dash Diet Side Dish Recipes

Rosemary Endives

Preparation time: 10 minutes
Cooking time: 20 minutes
Servings: 4

Ingredients:

- 2 endives, halved lengthwise
- 2 tablespoons olive oil
- 1 teaspoon rosemary, dried
- ½ teaspoon turmeric powder
- A pinch of black pepper

Directions:

1. In a baking pan, combine the endives with the oil and the other ingredients, toss gently, introduce in the oven and bake at 400 degrees F for 20 minutes.
2. Divide between plates and serve as a side dish.

Nutrition: calories 66, fat 7.1, fiber 1, carbs 1.2, protein 0.3

Lemony Endives

Preparation time: 10 minutes
Cooking time: 20 minutes
Servings: 4

Ingredients:
- 4 endives, halved lengthwise
- 1 tablespoon lemon juice
- 1 tablespoon lemon zest, grated
- 2 tablespoons fat-free parmesan, grated
- 2 tablespoons olive oil
- A pinch of black pepper

Directions:
1. In a baking dish, combine the endives with the lemon juice and the other ingredients except the parmesan and toss.
2. Sprinkle the parmesan on top, bake the endives at 400 degrees F for 20 minutes, divide between plates and serve as a side dish.

Nutrition: calories 71, fat 7.1, fiber 0.9, carbs 2.3, protein 0.9

Pesto Asparagus

Preparation time: 10 minutes
Cooking time: 20 minutes
Servings: 4

Ingredients:
- 1 pound asparagus, trimmed
- 2 tablespoons basil pesto
- 1 tablespoon lemon juice
- A pinch of black pepper
- 3 tablespoons olive oil
- 2 tablespoons cilantro, chopped

Directions:
1. Arrange the asparagus n a lined baking sheet, add the pesto and the other ingredients, toss, introduce in the oven and cook at 400 degrees F for 20 minutes.
2. Divide between plates and serve as a side dish.

Nutrition: calories 114, fat 10.7, fiber 2.4, carbs 4.6, protein 2.6

Paprika Carrots

Preparation time: 10 minutes
Cooking time: 30 minutes
Servings: 4

Ingredients:
- 1 pound baby carrots, trimmed
- 1 tablespoon sweet paprika
- 1 teaspoon lime juice
- 3 tablespoons olive oil
- A pinch of black pepper
- 1 teaspoon sesame seeds

Directions:
1. Arrange the carrots on a lined baking sheet, add the paprika and the other ingredients except the sesame seeds, toss, introduce in the oven and bake at 400 degrees F for 30 minutes.
2. Divide the carrots between plates, sprinkle sesame seeds on top and serve as a side dish.

Nutrition: calories 142, fat 11.3, fiber 4.1, carbs 11.4, protein 1.2

Creamy Potato Pan

Preparation time: 10 minutes
Cooking time: 1 hour
Servings: 8

Ingredients:

- 1 pound gold potatoes, peeled and cut into wedges
- 2 tablespoons olive oil
- 1 red onion, chopped
- 2 garlic cloves, minced
- 2 cups coconut cream
- 1 tablespoon thyme, chopped
- ¼ teaspoon nutmeg, ground
- ½ cup low-fat parmesan, grated

Directions:

1. Heat up a pan with the oil over medium heat, add the onion and the garlic and sauté for 5 minutes.
2. Add the potatoes and brown them for 5 minutes more.
3. Add the cream and the rest of the ingredients, toss gently, bring to a simmer and cook over medium heat for 40 minutes more.
4. Divide the mix between plates and serve as a side dish.

Nutrition: calories 230, fat 19.1, fiber 3.3, carbs 14.3, protein 3.6

Sesame Cabbage

Preparation time: 10 minutes
Cooking time: 20 minutes
Servings: 4

Ingredients:

- 1 pound green cabbage, roughly shredded
- 2 tablespoons olive oil
- A pinch of black pepper
- 1 shallot, chopped
- 2 garlic cloves, minced
- 2 tablespoons balsamic vinegar
- 2 teaspoons hot paprika
- 1 teaspoon sesame seeds

Directions:

1. Heat up a pan with the oil over medium heat, add the shallot and the garlic and sauté for 5 minutes.
2. Add the cabbage and the other ingredients, toss, cook over medium heat for 15 minutes, divide between plates and serve.

Nutrition: calories 101, fat 7.6, fiber 3.4, carbs 84, protein 1.9

Cilantro Broccoli

Preparation time: 10 minutes
Cooking time: 30 minutes
Servings: 4

Ingredients:

- 2 tablespoons olive oil
- 1 pound broccoli florets
- 2 garlic cloves, minced
- 2 tablespoons chili sauce
- 1 tablespoon lemon juice
- A pinch of black pepper
- 2 tablespoons cilantro, chopped

Directions:

1. In a baking pan, combine the broccoli with the oil, garlic and the other ingredients, toss a bit, introduce in the oven and bake at 400 degrees F for 30 minutes.
2. Divide the mix between plates and serve as a side dish.

Nutrition: calories 103, fat 7.4, fiber 3, carbs 8.3, protein 3.4

Chili Brussels Sprouts

Preparation time: 10 minutes
Cooking time: 25 minutes
Servings: 4

Ingredients:
- 1 tablespoon olive oil
- 1 pound Brussels sprouts, trimmed and halved
- 2 garlic cloves, minced
- ½ cup low-fat mozzarella, shredded
- A pinch of pepper flakes, crushed

Directions:
1. In a baking dish, combine the sprouts with the oil and the other ingredients except the cheese and toss.
2. Sprinkle the cheese on top, introduce in the oven and bake at 400 degrees F for 25 minutes.
3. Divide between plates and serve as a side dish.

Nutrition: calories 91, fat 4.5, fiber 4.3, carbs 10.9, protein 5

Brussels Sprouts and Green Onions Mix

Preparation time: 10 minutes
Cooking time: 25 minutes
Servings: 4

Ingredients:
- 2 tablespoons olive oil
- 1 pound Brussels sprouts, trimmed and halved
- 3 green onions, chopped
- 2 garlic cloves, minced
- 1 tablespoon balsamic vinegar
- 1 tablespoon sweet paprika
- A pinch of black pepper

Directions:
1. In a baking pan, combine the Brussels sprouts with the oil and the other ingredients, toss and bake at 400 degrees F for 25 minutes.
2. Divide the mix between plates and serve.

Nutrition: calories 121, fat 7.6, fiber 5.2, carbs 12.7, protein 4.4

Mashed Cauliflower

Preparation time: 10 minutes
Cooking time: 25 minutes
Servings: 4

Ingredients:

- 2 pounds cauliflower florets
- ½ cup coconut milk
- A pinch of black pepper
- ½ cup low-fat sour cream
- 1 tablespoon cilantro, chopped
- 1 tablespoon chives, chopped

Directions:

1. Put the cauliflower in a pot, add water to cover, bring to a boil over medium heat, cook for 25 minutes and drain.
2. Mash the cauliflower, add the milk, black pepper and the cream, whisk well, divide between plates, sprinkle the rest of the ingredients on top and serve.

Nutrition: calories 188, fat 13.4, fiber 6.4, carbs 15, protein 6.1

Avocado Salad

Preparation time: 5 minutes
Cooking time: 0 minutes
Servings: 4

Ingredients:

- 2 tablespoons olive oil
- 2 avocados, peeled, pitted and cut into wedges
- 1 cup kalamata olives, pitted and halved
- 1 cup tomatoes, cubed
- 1 tablespoon ginger, grated
- A pinch of black pepper
- 2 cups baby arugula
- 1 tablespoon balsamic vinegar

Directions:

1. In a bowl, combine the avocados with the kalamata and the other ingredients, toss and serve as a side dish.

Nutrition: calories 320, fat 30.4, fiber 8.7, carbs 13.9, protein 3

Radish Salad

Preparation time: 5 minutes
Cooking time: 0 minutes
Servings: 4

Ingredients:
- 2 green onions, sliced
- 1 pound radishes, cubed
- 2 tablespoons balsamic vinegar
- 2 tablespoon olive oil
- 1 teaspoon chili powder
- 1 cup black olives, pitted and halved
- A pinch of black pepper

Directions:
1. In a large salad bowl, combine radishes with the onions and the other ingredients, toss and serve as a side dish.

Nutrition: calories 123, fat 10.8, fiber 3.3, carbs 7, protein 1.3

Lemony Endives Salad

Preparation time: 5 minutes
Cooking time: 0 minutes
Servings: 4

Ingredients:
- 2 endives, roughly shredded
- 1 tablespoon dill, chopped
- ¼ cup lemon juice
- ¼ cup olive oil
- 2 cups baby spinach
- 2 tomatoes, cubed
- 1 cucumber, sliced
- ½ cups walnuts, chopped

Directions:
1. In a large bowl, combine the endives with the spinach and the other ingredients, toss and serve as a side dish.

Nutrition: calories 238, fat 22.3, fiber 3.1, carbs 8.4, protein 5.7

Olives and Corn Mix

Preparation time: 5 minutes
Cooking time: 0 minutes
Servings: 4

Ingredients:
- 2 tablespoons olive oil
- 1 tablespoon balsamic vinegar
- A pinch of black pepper
- 4 cups corn
- 2 cups black olives, pitted and halved
- 1 red onion, chopped
- ½ cup cherry tomatoes, halved
- 1 tablespoon basil, chopped
- 1 tablespoon jalapeno, chopped
- 2 cups romaine lettuce, shredded

Directions:
1. In a large bowl, combine the corn with the olives, lettuce and the other ingredients, toss well, divide between plates and serve as a side dish.

Nutrition: calories 290, fat 16.1, fiber 7.4, carbs 37.6, protein 6.2

Arugula and Pine Nuts Salad

Preparation time: 5 minutes
Cooking time: 0 minutes
Servings: 4

Ingredients:
- ¼ cup pomegranate seeds
- 5 cups baby arugula
- 6 tablespoons green onions, chopped
- 1 tablespoon balsamic vinegar
- 2 tablespoons olive oil
- 3 tablespoons pine nuts
- ½ shallot, chopped

Directions:
1. In a salad bowl, combine the arugula with the pomegranate and the other ingredients, toss and serve.

Nutrition: calories 120, fat 11.6, fiber 0.9, carbs 4.2, protein 1.8

Almonds and Spinach

Preparation time: 10 minutes
Cooking time: 0 minutes
Servings: 4

Ingredients:
- 2 tablespoons olive oil
- 2 avocados, peeled, pitted and cut into wedges
- 3 cups baby spinach
- ¼ cup almonds, toasted and chopped
- 1 tablespoon lemon juice
- 1 tablespoon cilantro, chopped

Directions:
1. In a bowl, combine the avocados with the almonds, spinach and the other ingredients, toss and serve as a side dish.

Nutrition: calories 181, fat 4, fiber 4.8, carbs 11.4, protein 6

Green Beans and Corn Salad

Preparation time: 4 minutes
Cooking time: 0 minutes
Servings: 4

Ingredients:

- Juice of 1 lime
- 2 cups romaine lettuce, shredded
- 1 cup corn
- ½ pound green beans, blanched and halved
- 1 cucumber, chopped
- 1/3 cup chives, chopped

Directions:

1. In a bowl, combine the green beans with the corn and the other ingredients, toss and serve.

Nutrition: calories 225, fat 12, fiber 2.4, carbs 11.2, protein 3.5

Endives and Kale Salad

Preparation time: 4 minutes
Cooking time: 0 minutes
Servings: 4

Ingredients:

- 3 tablespoons olive oil
- 2 endives, trimmed and shredded
- 2 tablespoons lime juice
- 1 tablespoon lime zest, grated
- 1 red onion, sliced
- 1 tablespoon balsamic vinegar
- 1 pound kale, torn
- A pinch of black pepper

Directions:

1. In a bowl, combine the endives with the kale and the other ingredients, toss well and serve cold as a side salad.

Nutrition: calories 270, fat 11.4, fiber 5, carbs 14.3, protein 5.7

Edamame Salad

Preparation time: 5 minutes
Cooking time: 6 minutes
Servings: 4

Ingredients:
- 2 tablespoons olive oil
- 2 tablespoons balsamic vinegar
- 2 garlic cloves, minced
- 3 cups edamame, shelled
- 1 tablespoon chives, chopped
- 2 shallots, chopped

Directions:
1. Heat up a pan with the oil over medium heat, add the edamame, the garlic and the other ingredients, toss, cook for 6 minutes, divide between plates and serve.

Nutrition: calories 270, fat 8.4, fiber 5.3, carbs 11.4, protein 6

Grapes and Avocados Salad

Preparation time: 5 minutes
Cooking time: 0 minutes
Servings: 4

Ingredients:
- 2 cups baby spinach
- 2 avocados, peeled, pitted and roughly cubed
- 1 cucumber, sliced
- 1 and ½ cups green grapes, halved
- 2 tablespoons avocado oil
- 1 tablespoon cider vinegar
- 2 tablespoons parsley, chopped
- A pinch of black pepper

Directions:
1. In a salad bowl, combine the baby spinach with the avocados and the other ingredients, toss and serve.

Nutrition: calories 277, fat 11.4, fiber 5, carbs 14.6, protein 4

Oregano Eggplant Mix

Preparation time: 10 minutes
Cooking time: 20 minutes
Servings: 4

Ingredients:
- 2 big eggplants, roughly cubed
- 1 tablespoon oregano, chopped
- ½ cup low-fat parmesan, grated
- ¼ teaspoon garlic powder
- 2 tablespoons olive oil
- A pinch of black pepper

Directions:
1. In a baking pan combine the eggplants with the oregano and the other ingredients except the cheese and toss.
2. Sprinkle parmesan on top, introduce in the oven and bake at 370 degrees F for 20 minutes.
3. Divide between plates and serve as a side dish.

Nutrition: calories 248, fat 8.4, fiber 4, carbs 14.3, protein 5.4

Baked Tomatoes Mix

Preparation time: 10 minutes
Cooking time: 20 minutes
Servings: 4

Ingredients:

- 2 pounds tomatoes, halved
- 1 tablespoon basil, chopped
- 3 tablespoons olive oil
- Zest of 1 lemon, grated
- 3 garlic cloves, minced
- ¼ cup low-fat parmesan, grated
- A pinch of black pepper

Directions:

1. In a baking pan, combine the tomatoes with the basil and the other ingredients except the cheese and toss.
2. Sprinkle the parmesan on top, introduce in the oven at 375 degrees F for 20 minutes, divide between plates and serve as a side dish.

Nutrition: calories 224, fat 12, fiber 4.3, carbs 10.8, protein 5.1

Thyme Mushrooms

Preparation time: 10 minutes
Cooking time: 30 minutes
Servings: 4

Ingredients:
- 2 pounds white mushrooms, halved
- 4 garlic cloves, minced
- 2 tablespoons olive oil
- 1 tablespoon thyme, chopped
- 2 tablespoons parsley, chopped
- Black pepper to the taste

Directions:
1. In a baking pan, combine the mushrooms with the garlic and the other ingredients, toss, introduce in the oven and cook at 400 degrees F for 30 minutes.
2. Divide between plates and serve as a side dish.

Nutrition: calories 251, fat 9.3, fiber 4, carbs 13.2, protein 6

Spinach and Corn Sauté

Preparation time: 10 minutes
Cooking time: 15 minutes
Servings: 4

Ingredients:
- 1 cup corn
- 1 pound spinach leaves
- 1 teaspoon sweet paprika
- 1 tablespoon olive oil
- 1 yellow onion, chopped
- ½ cup basil, torn
- A pinch of black pepper
- ½ teaspoon red pepper flakes

Directions:
1. Heat up a pan with the oil over medium-high heat, add the onion, stir and sauté for 5 minutes.
2. Add the corn, spinach and the other ingredients, toss, cook over medium heat for 10 minutes more, divide between plates and serve.

Nutrition: calories 201, fat 13.1, fiber 2.5, carbs 14.4, protein 3.7

Corn and Scallions Sauté

Preparation time: 10 minutes
Cooking time: 15 minutes
Servings: 4

Ingredients:

- 4 cups corn
- 1 tablespoon avocado oil
- 2 shallots, chopped
- 1 teaspoon chili powder
- 2 tablespoons tomato paste, no-salt-added
- 3 scallions, chopped
- A pinch of black pepper

Directions:

1. Heat up a pan with the oil over medium-high heat, add the scallions and chili powder, stir and sauté for 5 minutes.
2. Add the corn and the other ingredients, toss, cook for 10 minutes more, divide between plates and serve as a side dish.

Nutrition: calories 259, fat 11.1, fiber 2.6, carbs 13.2, protein 3.5

Spinach and Mango Salad

Preparation time: 10 minutes
Cooking time: 0 minutes
Servings: 4

Ingredients:
- 1 cup mango, peeled and cubed
- 4 cups baby spinach
- 1 tablespoon olive oil
- 2 spring onions, chopped
- 1 tablespoon lemon juice
- 1 tablespoon capers, drained, no-salt-added
- 1/3 cup almonds, chopped

Directions:
1. In a bowl, mix the spinach with the mango an d the other ingredients, toss and serve.

Nutrition: calories 200, fat 7.4, fiber 3, carbs 4.7, protein 4.4

Mustard Potatoes

Preparation time: 5 minutes
Cooking time: 1 hour
Servings: 4

Ingredients:

- 1 pound gold potatoes, peeled and cut into wedges
- 2 tablespoons olive oil
- A pinch of black pepper
- 2 tablespoons rosemary, chopped
- 1 tablespoon Dijon mustard
- 2 garlic cloves, minced

Directions:

1. In a baking pan, combine the potatoes with the oil and the other ingredients, toss, introduce in the oven at 400 degrees F and bake for about 1 hour.
2. Divide between plates and serve as a side dish right away.

Nutrition: calories 237, fat 11.5, fiber 6.4, carbs 14.2, protein 9

Coconut Brussels Sprouts

Preparation time: 5 minutes
Cooking time: 30 minutes
Servings: 4

Ingredients:

- 1 pound Brussels sprouts, trimmed and halved
- 1 cup coconut cream
- 1 tablespoon olive oil
- 2 shallots, chopped
- A pinch of black pepper
- ½ cup cashews, chopped

Directions:

1. In a roasting pan, combine the sprouts with the cream and the rest of the ingredients, toss, and bake in the oven for 30 minutes at 350 degrees F.
2. Divide between plates and serve as a side dish.

Nutrition: calories 270, fat 6.5, fiber 5.3, carbs 15.9, protein 3.4

Sage Carrots

Preparation time: 10 minutes
Cooking time: 30 minutes
Servings: 4

Ingredients:
- 2 tablespoons olive oil
- 2 teaspoons sweet paprika
- 1 pound carrots, peeled and roughly cubed
- 1 red onion, chopped
- 1 tablespoon sage, chopped
- A pinch of black pepper

Directions:
1. In a baking pan, combine the carrots with the oil and the other ingredients, toss and bake at 380 degrees F for 30 minutes.
2. Divide between plates and serve.

Nutrition: calories 200, fat 8.7, fiber 2.5, carbs 7.9, protein 4

Garlic Mushrooms and Corn

Preparation time: 10 minutes
Cooking time: 20 minutes
Servings: 4

Ingredients:
- 1 pound white mushrooms, halved
- 2 cups corn
- 2 tablespoons olive oil
- 4 garlic cloves, minced
- 1 cup canned tomatoes, no-salt-added, chopped
- A pinch of black pepper
- ½ teaspoon chili powder

Directions:
1. Heat up a pan with the oil over medium heat, add the mushrooms, garlic and the corn, stir and sauté for 10 minutes.
2. Add the rest of the ingredients, toss, cook over medium heat for 10 minutes more, divide between plates and serve.

Nutrition: calories 285, fat 13, fiber 2.2, carbs 14.6, protein 6.7.

Pesto Green Beans

Preparation time: 10 minutes
Cooking time: 15 minutes
Servings: 4

Ingredients:

- 2 tablespoons basil pesto
- 2 teaspoons sweet paprika
- 1 pound green beans, trimmed and halved
- Juice of 1 lemon
- 2 tablespoons olive oil
- 1 red onion, sliced
- A pinch of black pepper

Directions:

1. Heat up a pan with the oil over medium-high heat, add the onion, stir and sauté for 5 minutes.
2. Add the beans and the rest of the ingredients, toss, cook over medium heat fro 10 minutes, divide between plates and serve.

Nutrition: calories 280, fat 10, fiber 7.6, carbs 13.9, protein 4.7

Tarragon Tomatoes

Preparation time: 5 minutes
Cooking time: 0 minutes
Servings: 4

Ingredients:
- 1 and ½ tablespoon olive oil
- 1 pound tomatoes, cut into wedges
- 1 tablespoon lime juice
- 1 tablespoon lime zest, grated
- 2 tablespoons tarragon, chopped
- A pinch of black pepper

Directions:
1. In a bowl, combine the tomatoes with the other ingredients, toss and serve as a side salad.

Nutrition: calories 170, fat 4, fiber 2.1, carbs 11.8, proteins 6

Almond Beets

Preparation time: 10 minutes
Cooking time: 30 minutes
Servings: 4

Ingredients:
- 4 beets, peeled and cut into wedges
- 3 tablespoons olive oil
- 2 tablespoons almonds, chopped
- 2 tablespoons balsamic vinegar
- A pinch of black pepper
- 2 tablespoons parsley, chopped

Directions:
1. In a baking pan, combine the beets with the oil and the other ingredients, toss, introduce in the oven and bake at 400 degrees f for 30 minutes.
2. Divide the mix between plates and serve.

Nutrition: calories 230, fat 11, fiber 4.2, carbs 7.3, protein 3.6

Minty Tomatoes and Corn

Preparation time: 5 minutes
Cooking time: 0 minutes
Servings: 4

Ingredients:

- 2 tablespoons mint, chopped
- 1 pound tomatoes, cut into wedges
- 2 cups corn
- 2 tablespoons olive oil
- 1 tablespoon rosemary vinegar
- A pinch of black pepper

Directions:

1. In a salad bowl, combine the tomatoes with the corn and the other ingredients, toss and serve.

Enjoy!

Nutrition: calories 230, fat 7.2, fiber 2, carbs 11.6, protein 4

Zucchini and Avocado Salsa

Preparation time: 5 minutes
Cooking time: 10 minutes
Servings: 4

Ingredients:
- 2 tablespoons olive oil
- 2 zucchinis, cubed
- 1 avocado, peeled, pitted and cubed
- 2 tomatoes, cubed
- 1 cucumber, cubed
- 1 yellow onion, chopped
- 2 tablespoons fresh lime juice
- 2 tablespoons cilantro, chopped

Directions:
1. Heat up a pan with the oil over medium heat, add the onion and the zucchinis, toss and cook for 5 minutes.
2. Add the rest of the ingredients, toss, cook for 5 minutes more, divide between plates and serve.

Nutrition: calories 290, fat 11.2, fiber 6.1, carbs 14.7, protein 5.6

Apples and Cabbage Mix

Preparation time: 5 minutes
Cooking time: 0 minutes
Servings: 4

Ingredients:

- 2 green apples, cored and cubed
- 1 red cabbage head, shredded
- 2 tablespoons balsamic vinegar
- ½ teaspoon caraway seeds
- 2 tablespoons olive oil
- Black pepper to the taste

Directions:

1. In a bowl, combine the cabbage with the apples and the other ingredients, toss and serve as a side salad.

Nutrition: calories 165, fat 7.4, fiber 7.3, carbs 26, protein 2.6

Roasted Beets

Preparation time: 10 minutes
Cooking time: 30 minutes
Servings: 4

Ingredients:
- 4 beets, peeled and cut into wedges
- 2 tablespoons olive oil
- 2 garlic cloves, minced
- A pinch of black pepper
- ¼ cup parsley, chopped
- ¼ cup walnuts, chopped

Directions:
1. In a baking dish, combine the beets with the oil and the other ingredients, toss to coat, introduce in the oven at 420 degrees F, bake for 30 minutes, divide between plates and serve as a side dish.

Nutrition: calories 156, fat 11.8, fiber 2.7, carbs 11.5, protein 3.8

Dill Cabbage

Preparation time: 10 minutes
Cooking time: 15 minutes
Servings: 4

Ingredients:

- 1 pound green cabbage, shredded
- 1 yellow onion, chopped
- 1 tomato, cubed
- 1 tablespoon dill, chopped
- A pinch of black pepper
- 1 tablespoon olive oil

Directions:

1. Heat up a pan with the oil over medium heat, add the onion and sauté for 5 minutes.
2. Add the cabbage and the rest of the ingredients, toss, cook over medium heat for 10 minutes, divide between plates and serve.

Nutrition: calories 74, fat 3.7, fiber 3.7, carbs 10.2, protein 2.1

Cabbage and Carrot Salad

Preparation time: 5 minutes
Cooking time: 0 minutes
Servings: 4

Ingredients:
- 2 shallots, chopped
- 2 carrots, grated
- 1 big red cabbage head, shredded
- 1 tablespoon olive oil
- 1 tablespoon red vinegar
- A pinch of black pepper
- 1 tablespoon lime juice

Directions:
1. In a bowl, mix the cabbage with the shallots and the other ingredients, toss and serve as a side salad.

Nutrition: calories 106, fat 3.8, fiber 6.5, carbs 18, protein 3.3

Tomato and Olives Salsa

Preparation time: 10 minutes
Cooking time: 0 minutes
Servings: 6

Ingredients:

- 1 pound cherry tomatoes, halved
- 2 tablespoons olive oil
- 1 cup kalamata olives, pitted and halved
- A pinch of black pepper
- 1 red onion, chopped
- 1 tablespoon balsamic vinegar
- ¼ cup cilantro, chopped

Directions:

1. In a bowl, mix the tomatoes with the olives and the other ingredients, toss and serve as a side salad.

Nutrition: calories 131, fat 10.9, fiber 3.1, carbs 9.2, protein 1.6

Zucchini Salad

Preparation time: 4 minutes
Cooking time: 0 minutes
Servings: 4

Ingredients:
- 2 zucchinis, cut with a spiralizer
- 1 red onion, sliced
- 1 tablespoon basil pesto
- 1 tablespoon lemon juice
- 1 tablespoon olive oil
- ½ cup cilantro, chopped
- Black pepper to the taste

Directions:
1. In a salad bowl, mix the zucchinis with the onion and the other ingredients, toss and serve.

Nutrition: calories 58, fat 3.8, fiber 1.8, carbs 6, protein 1.6

Curry Carrots Slaw

Preparation time: 4 minutes
Cooking time: 0 minutes
Servings: 4

Ingredients:
- 1 pound carrots, peeled and roughly grated
- 2 tablespoons avocado oil
- 2 tablespoons lemon juice
- 3 tablespoons sesame seeds
- ½ teaspoon curry powder
- 1 teaspoon rosemary, dried
- ½ teaspoon cumin, ground

Directions:
1. In a bowl, mix the carrots with the oil, lemon juice and the other ingredients, toss and serve cold as a side salad.

Nutrition: calories 99, fat 4.4, fiber 4.2, carbs 13.7, protein 2.4

Lettuce and Beet Salad

Preparation time: 5 minutes
Cooking time: 0 minutes
Servings: 4

Ingredients:
- 1 tablespoon ginger, grated
- 2 garlic cloves, minced
- 4 cups romaine lettuce, torn
- 1 beet, peeled and grated
- 2 green onions, chopped
- 1 tablespoon balsamic vinegar
- 1 tablespoon sesame seeds

Directions:
1. In a bowl, combine the lettuce with the ginger, garlic and the other ingredients, toss and serve as a side dish.

Nutrition: calories 42, fat 1.4, fiber 1.5, carbs 6.7, protein 1.4

Herbed Radishes

Preparation time: 5 minutes
Cooking time: 0 minutes
Servings: 4

Ingredients:
- 1 pound red radishes, roughly cubed
- 1 tablespoon chives, chopped
- 1 tablespoon parsley, chopped
- 1 tablespoon oregano, chopped
- 2 tablespoons olive oil
- 1 tablespoon lime juice
- Black pepper to the taste

Directions:
1. In a salad bowl, mix the radishes with the chives and the other ingredients, toss and serve.

Nutrition: calories 85, fat 7.3, fiber 2.4, carbs 5.6, protein 1

Baked Fennel Mix

Preparation time: 5 minutes
Cooking time: 20 minutes
Servings: 4

Ingredients:
- 2 fennel bulbs, sliced
- 1 teaspoon sweet paprika
- 1 small red onion, sliced
- 2 tablespoons olive oil
- 2 tablespoons lime juice
- 2 tablespoons dill, chopped
- Black pepper to the taste

Directions:
1. In a roasting pan, combine the fennel with the paprika and the other ingredients, toss, and bake at 380 degrees F for 20 minutes.
2. Divide the mix between plates and serve.

Nutrition: calories 114, fat 7.4, fiber 4.5, carbs 13.2, protein 2.1

Roasted Peppers

Preparation time: 10 minutes
Cooking time: 30 minutes
Servings: 4

Ingredients:
- 1 pound mixed bell peppers, cut into wedges
- 1 red onion, thinly sliced
- 2 tablespoons olive oil
- Black pepper to the taste
- 1 tablespoon oregano, chopped
- 2 tablespoons mint leaves, chopped

Directions:
1. In a roasting pan, combine the bell peppers with the onion and the other ingredients, toss and bake at 380 degrees F for 30 minutes.
2. Divide the mix between plates and serve.

Nutrition: calories 240, fat 8.2, fiber 4.2, carbs 11.3, protein 5.6

Dates and Cabbage Sauté

Preparation time: 5 minutes
Cooking time: 15 minutes
Servings: 4

Ingredients:

- 1 pound red cabbage, shredded
- 8 dates, pitted and sliced
- 2 tablespoons olive oil
- ¼ cup low-sodium veggie stock
- 2 tablespoons chives, chopped
- 2 tablespoons lemon juice
- Black pepper to the taste

Directions:

1. Heat up a pan with the oil over medium heat, add the cabbage and the dates, toss and cook for 4 minutes.
2. Add the stock and the other ingredients, toss, cook over medium heat for 11 minutes more, divide between plates and serve.

Nutrition: calories 280, fat 8.1, fiber 4.1, carbs 8.7, protein 6.3

Black Beans Mix

Preparation time: 4 minutes
Cooking time: 0 minutes
Servings: 4

Ingredients:
- 3 cups canned black beans, no-salt-added, drained and rinsed
- 1 cup cherry tomatoes, halved
- 2 shallots, chopped
- 3 tablespoons olive oil
- 1 tablespoon balsamic vinegar
- Black pepper to the taste
- 1 tablespoon chives, chopped

Directions:
1. In a bowl, combine the beans with the tomatoes and the other ingredients, toss and serve cold as a side dish.

Nutrition: calories 310, fat 11.0, fiber 5.3, carbs 19.6, protein 6.8

Olives and Endives Mix

Preparation time: 4 minutes
Cooking time: 0 minutes
Servings: 4

Ingredients:
- 2 spring onions, chopped
- 2 endives, shredded
- 1 cup black olives, pitted and sliced
- ½ cup kalamata olives, pitted and sliced
- ¼ cup apple cider vinegar
- 2 tablespoons olive oil
- 1 tablespoons cilantro, chopped

Directions:
1. In a bowl, mix the endives with the olives and the other ingredients, toss and serve.

Nutrition: calories 230, fat 9.1, fiber 6.3, carbs 14.6, protein 7.2

Tomatoes and Cucumber Salad

Preparation time: 5 minutes
Cooking time: 0 minutes
Servings: 4

Ingredients:
- ½ pound tomatoes, cubed
- 2 cucumber, sliced
- 1 tablespoon olive oil
- 2 spring onions, chopped
- Black pepper to the taste
- Juice of 1 lime
- ½ cup basil, chopped

Directions:
1. In a salad bowl, combine the tomatoes with the cucumber and the other ingredients, toss and serve cold.

Nutrition: calories 224, fat 11.2, fiber 5.1, carbs 8.9, protein 6.2

Peppers and Carrot Salad

Preparation time: 5 minutes
Cooking time: 0 minutes
Servings: 4

Ingredients:

- 1 cup cherry tomatoes, halved
- 1 yellow bell pepper, chopped
- 1 red bell pepper, chopped
- 1 green bell pepper, chopped
- ½ pound carrots, shredded
- 3 tablespoons red wine vinegar
- 2 tablespoons olive oil
- 1 tablespoon cilantro, chopped
- Black pepper to the taste

Directions:

1. In a salad bowl, mix the tomatoes with the peppers, carrots and the other ingredients, toss and serve as a side salad.

Nutrition: calories 123, fat 4, fiber 8.4, carbs 14.4, protein 1.1

Black Beans and Rice Mix

Preparation time: 10 minutes
Cooking time: 30 minutes
Servings: 4

Ingredients:
- 2 tablespoons olive oil
- 1 yellow onion, chopped
- 1 cup canned black beans, no-salt-added, drained and rinsed
- 2 cup black rice
- 4 cups low-sodium chicken stock
- 2 tablespoons thyme, chopped
- Zest of ½ lemon, grated
- A pinch of black pepper

Directions:
1. Heat up a pan with the oil over medium-high heat, add the onion, stir and sauté for 4 minutes.
2. Add the beans, rice and the other ingredients, toss, bring to a boil and cook over medium heat for 25 minutes.
3. Stir the mix, divide between plates and serve.

Nutrition: calories 290, fat 15.3, fiber 6.2, carbs 14.6, protein 8

Rice and Cauliflower Mix

Preparation time: 10 minutes
Cooking time: 25 minutes
Servings: 4

Ingredients:
- 1 cup cauliflower florets
- 1 cup white rice
- 2 cups low-sodium chicken stock
- 1 tablespoon avocado oil
- 2 shallots, chopped
- ¼ cup cranberries
- ½ cup almonds, sliced

Directions:
1. Heat up a pan with the oil over medium heat, add the shallots, stir and sauté for 5 minutes.
2. Add the cauliflower, the rice and the other ingredients, toss, bring to a simmer and cook over medium heat for 20 minutes.
3. Divide the mix between plates and serve.

Nutrition: calories 290, fat 15.1, fiber 5.6, carbs 7, protein 4.5

Balsamic Beans Mix

Preparation time: 10 minutes
Cooking time: 0 minutes
Servings: 4

Ingredients:

- 2 cups canned black beans, no-salt-added, drained and rinsed
- 2 cups canned white beans, no-salt-added, drained and rinsed
- 2 tablespoons balsamic vinegar
- 2 tablespoons olive oil
- 1 teaspoon oregano, dried
- 1 teaspoon basil, dried
- 1 tablespoon chives, chopped

Directions:

1. In a salad bowl, combine the beans with the vinegar and the other ingredients, toss and serve as a side salad.

Nutrition: calories 322, fat 15.1, fiber 10, carbs 22.0, protein 7

Creamy Beets

Preparation time: 5 minutes
Cooking time: 20 minutes
Servings: 4

Ingredients:
- 1 pound beets, peeled and cubed
- 1 red onion, chopped
- 1 tablespoon olive oil
- ½ cup coconut cream
- 4 tablespoons non-fat yogurt
- 1 tablespoon chives, chopped

Directions:
1. Heat up a pan with the oil over medium heat, add the onion, stir and sauté for 4 minutes.
2. Add the beets, cream and the other ingredients, toss, cook over medium heat for 15 minutes more, divide between plates and serve.

Nutrition: calories 250, fat 13.4, fiber 3, carbs 13.3, protein 6.4

Avocado and Bell Peppers Mix

Preparation time: 10 minutes
Cooking time: 14 minutes
Servings: 4

Ingredients:
- 1 tablespoon avocado oil
- 1 teaspoon sweet paprika
- 1 pound mixed bell peppers, cut into strips
- 1 avocado, peeled, pitted and halved
- 1 teaspoon garlic powder
- 1 teaspoon rosemary, dried
- ½ cup low-sodium veggie stock
- Black pepper to the taste

Directions:
1. Heat up a pan with the oil over medium-high heat, add all the bell peppers, stir and sauté for 5 minutes.
2. Add the rest of the ingredients, toss, cook for 9 minutes more over medium heat, divide between plates and serve.

Nutrition: calories 245, fat 13.8, fiber 5, carbs 22.5, protein 5.4

Roasted Sweet Potato and Beets

Preparation time: 10 minutes
Cooking time: 1 hour
Servings: 4

Ingredients:
- 3 tablespoons olive oil
- 2 sweet potatoes, peeled and cut into wedges
- 2 beets, peeled, and cut into wedges
- 1 tablespoon oregano, chopped
- 1 tablespoon lime juice
- Black pepper to the taste

Directions:
1. Arrange the sweet potatoes and the beets on a lined baking sheet, add the rest of the ingredients, toss, introduce in the oven and bake at 375 degrees F for 1 hour/
2. Divide between plates and serve as a side dish.

Nutrition: calories 240, fat 11.2, fiber 4, carbs 8.6, protein 12.1

Kale Sauté

Preparation time: 10 minutes
Cooking time: 15 minutes
Servings: 4

Ingredients:
- 2 tablespoons olive oil
- 3 tablespoons coconut aminos
- 1 pound kale, torn
- 1 red onion, chopped
- 2 garlic cloves, minced
- 1 tablespoon lime juice
- 1 tablespoon cilantro, chopped

Directions:
1. Heat up a pan with the olive oil over medium heat, add the onion and the garlic and sauté for 5 minutes.
2. Add the kale and the other ingredients, toss, cook over medium heat for 10 minutes, divide between plates and serve.

Nutrition: calories 200, fat 7.1, fiber 2, carbs 6.4, protein 6

Spiced Carrots

Preparation time: 10 minutes
Cooking time: 20 minutes
Servings: 4

Ingredients:
- 1 tablespoon lemon juice
- 1 tablespoon olive oil
- ½ teaspoon allspice, ground
- ½ teaspoon cumin, ground
- ½ teaspoon nutmeg, ground
- 1 pound baby carrots, trimmed
- 1 tablespoon rosemary, chopped
- Black pepper to the taste

Directions:
1. In a roasting pan, combine the carrots with the lemon juice, oil and the other ingredients, toss, introduce in the oven and bake at 400 degrees F for 20 minutes.
2. Divide between plates and serve.

Nutrition: calories 260, fat 11.2, fiber 4.5, carbs 8.3, protein 4.3

Lemony Artichokes

Preparation time: 10 minutes
Cooking time: 20 minutes
Servings: 4

Ingredients:
- 2 tablespoons lemon juice
- 4 artichokes, trimmed and halved
- 1 tablespoon dill, chopped
- 2 tablespoons olive oil
- A pinch of black pepper

Directions:
1. In a roasting pan, combine the artichokes with the lemon juice and the other ingredients, toss gently and bake at 400 degrees F for 20 minutes.
   Divide between plates and serve.

Nutrition: calories 140, fat 7.3, fiber 8.9, carbs 17.7, protein 5.5

Broccoli, Beans and Rice

Preparation time: 10 minutes
Cooking time: 30 minutes
Servings: 4

Ingredients:
- 1 cup broccoli florets, chopped
- 1 cup canned black beans, no-salt-added, drained
- 1 cup white rice
- 2 cups low-sodium chicken stock
- 2 teaspoons sweet paprika
- Black pepper to the taste

Directions:
1. Put the stock in a pot, heat up over medium heat, add the rice and the other ingredients, toss, bring to a boil and cook for 30 minutes stirring from time to time.
2. Divide the mix between plates and serve as a side dish.

Nutrition: calories 347, fat 1.2, fiber 9, carbs 69.3, protein 15.1

Baked Squash Mix

Preparation time: 10 minutes
Cooking time: 45 minutes
Servings: 4

Ingredients:
- 2 tablespoons olive oil
- 2 pounds butternut squash, peeled, and cut into wedges
- 1 tablespoon lemon juice
- 1 teaspoon chili powder
- 1 teaspoon garlic powder
- 2 teaspoons cilantro, chopped
- A pinch of black pepper

Directions
1. In a roasting pan, combine the squash with the oil and the other ingredients, toss gently, bake in the oven at 400 degrees F for 45 minutes, divide between plates and serve as a side dish.

Nutrition: calories 167, fat 7.4, fiber 4.9, carbs 27.5, protein 2.5

Creamy Asparagus

Preparation time: 5 minutes
Cooking time: 20 minutes
Servings: 4

Ingredients:
- ½ teaspoon nutmeg, ground
- 1 pound asparagus, trimmed and halved
- 1 cup coconut cream
- 1 yellow onion, chopped
- 2 tablespoons olive oil
- 1 tablespoon lime juice
- 1 tablespoon cilantro, chopped

Directions:
1. Heat up a pan with the oil over medium heat, add the onion and the nutmeg, stir and sauté for 5 minutes.
2. Add the asparagus and the other ingredients, toss, bring to a simmer and cook over medium heat for 15 minutes.
3. Divide between plates and serve.

Nutrition: calories 236, fat 21.6, fiber 4.4, carbs 11.4, protein 4.2

Basil Turnips Mix

Preparation time: 10 minutes
Cooking time: 15 minutes
Servings: 4

Ingredients:

- 1 tablespoon avocado oil
- 4 turnips, sliced
- ¼ cup basil, chopped
- Black pepper to the taste
- ¼ cup low-sodium veggie stock
- ½ cup walnuts, chopped
- 2 garlic cloves, minced

Directions:

1. Heat up a pan with the oil over medium-high heat, add the garlic and the turnips and brown for 5 minutes.
2. Add the rest of the ingredients, toss, cook for 10 minutes more, divide between plates and serve.

Nutrition: calories 140, fat 9.7, fiber 3.3, carbs 10.5, protein 5

Rice and Capers Mix

Preparation time: 10 minutes
Cooking time: 20 minutes
Servings: 4

Ingredients:

- 1 cup white rice
- 1 tablespoon capers, chopped
- 2 cups low-sodium chicken stock
- 1 red onion, chopped
- 1 tablespoon avocado oil
- 1 tablespoon cilantro, chopped
- 1 teaspoon sweet paprika

Directions:

1. Heat up a pan with the oil over medium-high heat, add the onion, stir and sauté for 5 minutes.
2. Add the rice, capers and the other ingredients, toss, bring to a simmer and cook for 15 minutes.
3. Divide the mix between plates and serve as a side dish.

Nutrition: calories 189, fat 0.9, fiber 1.6, carbs 40.2, protein 4.3

Spinach and Kale Mix

Preparation time: 5 minutes
Cooking time: 15 minutes
Servings: 4

Ingredients:
- 2 cups baby spinach
- 5 cups kale, torn
- 2 shallots, chopped
- 2 garlic cloves, minced
- 1 cup canned tomatoes, no-salt-added, chopped
- 1 tablespoon olive oil

Directions:
1. Heat up a pan with the oil over medium-high heat, add the shallots, stir and sauté for 5 minutes.
2. Add the spinach, kale and the other ingredients, toss, cook for 10 minutes more, divide between plates and serve as a side dish.

Nutrition: calories 89, fat 3.7, fiber 2.2, carbs 12.4, protein 3.6